Table Of Content s

Chapter 1: Understanding Addiction in Children

The Basics of Addiction

As parents, we all want the best for our children. We want to protect them, guide them, and provide them with a safe and secure future. However, in today's world, there are many challenges that our kids may face, and one of the most prevalent and dangerous is addiction.

In this subchapter, we will delve into the basics of addiction and provide you with essential information to help you understand this complex issue. By gaining a deeper understanding of addiction, you will be better equipped to prevent it in your children and support them if they are already struggling.

Addiction is a chronic disease that affects the brain and behavior. It is characterized by an intense craving for a substance or an activity, despite harmful consequences. It can manifest in various forms, including substance abuse, gaming addiction, or even excessive social media use. Understanding that addiction is a disease and not a moral failing is crucial in addressing and preventing it.

One of the key factors in raising a child who is less likely to develop an addiction is creating a nurturing and supportive environment. We will discuss strategies to build resilience in your child, such as fostering open communication, setting clear boundaries, and encouraging healthy coping mechanisms.

In addition to prevention, we will also explore how to support a loved one through addiction recovery. Recovery is a challenging journey, and as parents, your love and support can make a significant difference in their success.

Furthermore, we will touch upon nurturing a child with a predisposition to addiction. Genetics play a role in addiction, and being aware of your child's vulnerability can help you take proactive measures to keep them safe.

Raising awareness about addiction and prevention in children is essential not only for your own family but for the community as well. We will provide you with resources and tools to educate others, engage with schools and community organizations, and advocate for addiction prevention.

By understanding the basics of addiction, you will be able to protect your child's future and equip them with the knowledge and skills they need to make healthy choices. Together, let's create a generation of kids who are resilient, informed, and empowered to live a life free from the grips of addiction.

Common Risk Factors for Addiction in Children

As parents, we all want the best for our children. We strive to protect them from harm and set them on a path towards a bright future. However, when it comes to addiction, it can be challenging to identify the common risk factors that may put our children at risk. In this subchapter, we will explore these risk factors and equip you with the knowledge and tools to protect your child from addiction.

1. Genetics and Family History: Research has shown that addiction can run in families. If you or your partner have a history of substance abuse, your child may be more susceptible to developing an addiction. Understanding this genetic predisposition is crucial in taking proactive steps to prevent addiction in your child.

2. Childhood Trauma: Traumatic experiences during childhood, such as abuse, neglect, or witnessing domestic violence, can have a profound impact on a child's development. These adverse experiences can increase the likelihood of turning to substances as a coping mechanism later in life. As parents, it is vital to create a safe and nurturing environment for your child, ensuring their emotional well-being.

3. Peer Influence: As children grow older, their friends play an increasingly significant role in their lives. Peer pressure can be a powerful force, especially when it comes to experimenting with drugs or alcohol. Encouraging open communication and teaching your child about making healthy choices can help them resist negative peer influences.

4. Mental Health Disorders: Children with mental health disorders, such as anxiety, depression, or ADHD, may be more vulnerable to addiction. These disorders can increase the risk of self-medication with drugs or alcohol. Recognizing and addressing any underlying mental health issues in your child is essential in preventing addiction.

5. Lack of Parental Involvement: Parental involvement and monitoring play a vital role in addiction prevention. Children who lack parental guidance and supervision are more likely to engage in risky behaviors, including substance abuse. Stay actively involved in your child's life, set clear boundaries, and establish open lines of communication.

By understanding these common risk factors, you can take proactive steps to protect your child from addiction. Educate yourself about addiction prevention strategies, seek professional help if needed, and create a supportive and nurturing environment for your child.

Remember, early intervention and open communication are key in raising a resilient and addiction-free child.

In the following chapters, we will delve deeper into each risk factor, providing practical tips and strategies to mitigate these risks and safeguard your child's future. Together, we can make a difference in our children's lives and ensure a brighter, addiction-free future for them.

Recognizing Early Signs of Substance Abuse

As parents of young children, it is essential to be aware of the early signs of substance abuse. By familiarizing ourselves with these signs, we can intervene early and prevent our children from falling into the dangerous trap of addiction. In this subchapter, we will discuss the various indicators that may suggest a child is experimenting with or using substances. By recognizing these signs, we can take proactive measures to protect our children's future.

One of the first signs to look out for is a sudden change in behavior. If your child becomes increasingly secretive, withdrawn, or displays mood swings, it could be an indication of substance abuse. Pay attention to any significant changes in their academic performance, loss of interest in activities they once enjoyed, or a sudden change in their social circle.

Physical signs can also be indicative of substance abuse. Keep an eye out for bloodshot eyes, dilated or constricted pupils, unexplained weight loss or gain, frequent nosebleeds, or changes in sleeping patterns. These physical changes may be a result of drug or alcohol abuse.

Another red flag to watch for is a decline in personal hygiene and appearance. Substance abuse can lead to neglect of personal care, resulting in unkempt hair, body odor, and a lack of interest in grooming.

Changes in appetite can also be an early warning sign. Look for sudden and drastic changes in eating patterns, such as loss of appetite or binge eating. Substance abuse can have a significant impact on a child's overall health and well-being.

If you suspect your child may be experimenting with substances, it is crucial to open up a dialogue with them. Approach the conversation with empathy, understanding, and without judgment. Encourage open communication and assure them that you are there to support and help them through any challenges they may be facing.

Remember, early intervention is key. By recognizing the early signs of substance abuse, you can take the necessary steps to protect your child's future. Stay vigilant, foster a trusting relationship with your child, and educate yourself about addiction prevention. Together, we can raise awareness about addiction and ensure the well-being of our children.

Effects of Addiction on Child Development

Addiction is a complex and devastating disease that not only affects the individual struggling with it but also has profound consequences for their loved ones, especially children. In this subchapter, we will explore the various effects of addiction on child development and how parents can protect their children from the harmful impacts of this disease.

Children of parents with addiction face unique challenges that can significantly impact their emotional, physical, and cognitive development. Witnessing erratic behavior, neglect, or even abuse associated with addiction can lead to increased levels of stress and anxiety in children. These adverse experiences can disrupt healthy brain development, hinder academic performance, and impair social and emotional skills.

Furthermore, growing up in an environment where addiction is present can increase a child's risk of developing substance abuse problems in the future. Research has shown that children of addicts are more likely to experiment with drugs and alcohol themselves, perpetuating the cycle of addiction from one generation to the next. Therefore, it is crucial for parents to be aware of their own behaviors and take proactive steps to prevent addiction in their children.

Parenting a child with a predisposition to addiction requires a nurturing and supportive approach. Understanding the genetic and environmental factors that contribute to addiction can help parents create a protective and resilient environment for their children. Open and honest communication about the risks and consequences of substance abuse, coupled with setting clear boundaries and expectations, can help reduce the likelihood of addiction in vulnerable children.

For parents who are currently supporting a loved one through addiction recovery, it is essential to recognize the impact this process can have on their children. Children may experience feelings of guilt, shame, or confusion as they witness their loved one's struggle with addiction. Providing age-appropriate explanations, reassurance, and access to support services can help children cope with these challenging emotions and maintain a sense of stability.

Raising awareness about addiction and prevention in children is a shared responsibility of parents, communities, and schools. By educating ourselves and our children about the dangers of substance abuse, we can empower them to make healthy choices and resist peer pressure. Additionally, promoting positive coping mechanisms, such as sports, hobbies, and creative outlets, can help children develop resilience and avoid turning to substances as a way to cope with stress or emotional pain.

In conclusion, addiction can have far-reaching effects on child development. It is imperative for parents to recognize the significant impact addiction can have on their children and take proactive steps to protect them. By fostering a supportive and resilient environment, promoting open communication, and raising awareness about addiction prevention, parents can safeguard their children's future and break the cycle of addiction.

Chapter 2: How to Raise an Addict

Understanding Enabling Behaviors

Enabling behaviors are actions or behaviors that inadvertently support and perpetuate addictive behaviors in our children. As parents, it is crucial to recognize and understand these enabling behaviors in order to prevent addiction in our kids. By addressing these behaviors early on, we can create a safe and supportive environment that promotes healthy choices and reduces the risk of substance abuse.

Enabling behaviors can take many forms, and they often stem from a place of love and concern for our children. However, it is important to remember that enabling behaviors can inadvertently hinder their growth and perpetuate addictive patterns. Here are some common enabling behaviors to be aware of:

1. Denial: Denying or downplaying the severity of a problem can prevent us from taking necessary action. It is essential to acknowledge and address any signs of substance abuse or addictive behaviors early on.

2. Making Excuses: Covering up or making excuses for our child's actions or behaviors can enable them to continue down a destructive path. It is important to hold them accountable for their actions and set clear boundaries.

3. Financial Support: Providing unlimited financial support without any accountability can enable our children to fuel their addiction. It is crucial to establish boundaries and encourage financial independence.

4. Rescuing: Constantly rescuing our children from the consequences of their actions can prevent them from learning important life lessons. Allowing them to experience the natural consequences of their choices can be a powerful motivator for change.

5. Enabling Relationships: Allowing our children to associate with peers who engage in substance abuse or unhealthy behaviors can further enable their addiction. Encouraging positive friendships and setting limits on unhealthy relationships is vital.

Understanding enabling behaviors is the first step in preventing addiction in our children. By addressing these behaviors and creating a supportive environment, we can help our children make healthy choices and reduce their risk of substance abuse.

As parents, it is crucial to educate ourselves on addiction prevention and stay informed about current research and best practices. By nurturing open and honest communication with our children, we can create a safe space for them to talk about their feelings, fears, and challenges. By fostering resilience and emotional intelligence, we can empower our children to make healthy choices and navigate the challenges they may face throughout their lives.

Remember, addiction prevention starts early. By recognizing and addressing enabling behaviors, we can protect our children's future and provide them with the tools they need to lead healthy, fulfilling lives.

Setting Healthy Boundaries

One of the most crucial aspects of addiction prevention in children is setting healthy boundaries. As parents of young kids, it is essential to establish clear guidelines and limits that help protect them from the dangers of substance abuse. By doing so, we can create a safe and nurturing environment that supports their healthy development and reduces the risk of addiction. In this subchapter, we will explore effective strategies for setting boundaries and maintaining them throughout your child's life.

First and foremost, it is important to communicate openly with your children about the risks associated with substance abuse. Educate them about the dangers of drugs and alcohol in an age-appropriate manner, helping them understand the potential consequences and long-term effects. By providing them with accurate information, you empower them to make informed decisions and resist peer pressure.

Setting boundaries also involves establishing rules and expectations within your household. Clearly define what behaviors are acceptable and what is off-limits. Consistency is key here, as children need clear guidelines to understand the boundaries. Be firm but fair when enforcing these rules, ensuring that consequences are appropriate and consistent.

It is equally important to encourage open and honest communication within your family. Create a safe space where your children feel comfortable discussing their feelings, concerns, and experiences. By fostering a strong parent-child relationship built on trust, you can better understand any potential issues and address them promptly.

When parenting a teen with substance abuse problems, setting boundaries becomes even more crucial. Adolescence is a period of experimentation and curiosity, making it essential to establish clear limits to protect them from harm. Monitor their activities, including their social media and online presence, while respecting their privacy. Encourage healthy peer relationships and engage in open conversations about the dangers of substance abuse.

Supporting a loved one through addiction recovery requires a delicate balance of setting boundaries and providing support. Establish clear expectations for their behavior and hold them accountable for their actions. However, also offer empathy, understanding, and encouragement as they navigate their recovery journey. Seek professional help and involve support groups to ensure their successful recovery.

Lastly, nurturing a child with a predisposition to addiction requires a proactive approach to setting boundaries. Educate yourself about addiction and its genetic factors, allowing you to identify potential warning signs early on. Establish a supportive environment, focusing on building resilience, self-esteem, and healthy coping mechanisms. Encourage involvement in activities that promote physical and emotional well-being.

In conclusion, setting healthy boundaries is a vital component of addiction prevention in children. By establishing clear guidelines, fostering open communication, and providing support, parents can create a safe and nurturing environment that reduces the risk of substance abuse. Remember that each child is unique, and it is crucial to adapt your approach to their individual needs. By setting healthy boundaries, you are protecting their future and equipping them with the tools they need to make healthy choices.

Teaching Coping Skills and Emotional Regulation

One of the most important aspects of protecting our children from addiction is equipping them with the necessary coping skills and emotional regulation techniques. In today's fast-paced, high-pressure world, it is crucial that parents take an active role in teaching their young kids how to navigate their emotions and cope with stress in healthy ways. This subchapter will provide practical strategies and guidance for parents on how to effectively teach coping skills and emotional regulation to their children.

Coping skills are essential tools that help children manage their emotions and deal with challenging situations. By teaching our kids these skills, we can empower them to handle stress, peer pressure, and other triggers that may lead to substance abuse later in life. Some effective coping strategies include deep breathing exercises, journaling, engaging in physical activities, practicing mindfulness, and seeking support from trusted adults or friends.

Emotional regulation, on the other hand, refers to the ability to manage and express emotions in a healthy manner. Children who struggle with emotional regulation are more susceptible to turning to substances as a means of escape or self-medication. Parents can teach their kids how to identify and label their emotions, understand the triggers that lead to certain emotions, and find appropriate ways to express and cope with them. This can be done through open and honest communication, validating their feelings, and teaching problem-solving skills.

Incorporating these teachings into daily routines and activities is critical. Parents can create a safe and supportive environment where children feel comfortable expressing their emotions without fear of judgment or punishment. By modeling healthy coping skills and emotional regulation techniques, parents can effectively guide their children towards making positive choices.

Additionally, parents should be aware of their child's individual predisposition to addiction. If there is a family history of addiction or if a child exhibits certain risk factors, such as low self-esteem or impulsivity, it is even more important to focus on teaching coping skills and emotional regulation. By nurturing their child's emotional well-being and providing a strong support system, parents can help mitigate the risk of addiction.

Teaching coping skills and emotional regulation is an ongoing process that requires patience, consistency, and understanding. This subchapter aims to provide parents with practical tools and strategies to empower their children to make healthy choices and protect them from the dangers of addiction. By equipping our young kids with these essential skills, we can lay a solid foundation for their future well-being and resilience.

Promoting Open Communication

In the journey of raising our children, one of the most important aspects is fostering open and honest communication. As parents, we play a vital role in creating an environment where our children feel comfortable expressing their thoughts, feelings, and concerns. This subchapter focuses on the significance of promoting open communication as a means to prevent addiction in our kids.

Effective communication serves as a powerful tool in raising awareness about addiction and prevention in children. By establishing a safe and non-judgmental space, we can encourage our kids to openly discuss their feelings and experiences. It is essential to actively listen to our children, validating their emotions and offering guidance when necessary. Through open dialogue, we can gain insights into their lives, understand their struggles, and address any potential risks.

For parents who are navigating the challenges of parenting a teenager with substance abuse problems, open communication becomes even more crucial. Establishing trust and maintaining open lines of communication can help bridge the gap between parent and child. It is essential to create an atmosphere where teens feel comfortable discussing their concerns, experiences, and temptations. By fostering honest conversations, we can provide support, guidance, and intervention when needed, helping our teenagers overcome substance abuse challenges.

Supporting a loved one through addiction recovery requires a strong foundation of open communication. By creating an environment where individuals feel safe discussing their struggles and progress, we can offer unwavering support. Encouraging open communication during recovery not only helps in building trust but also provides an opportunity for family members to understand the challenges faced by their loved ones and offer much-needed empathy and encouragement.

Nurturing a child with a predisposition to addiction requires a delicate balance of open communication and proactive prevention. By engaging in age-appropriate conversations about the risks and consequences of substance abuse, we can equip our children with the necessary knowledge and skills to make informed decisions. Open communication fosters a strong parent-child relationship, enabling parents to guide and support their children through potential challenges.

In conclusion, promoting open communication is a fundamental aspect of addiction prevention in children. By creating an environment where our children feel safe expressing themselves, we can actively address their concerns, support them through challenges, and equip them with valuable tools to make healthy choices.

Open communication is the key to raising awareness about addiction, parenting teens with substance abuse problems, supporting loved ones in recovery, nurturing children with a predisposition to addiction, and ultimately protecting their future.

Seeking Professional Help for Early Intervention

In the journey of parenting, there may come a time when we face challenges that we never anticipated. One such challenge is dealing with addiction in our children. As parents, it is crucial that we recognize the signs and symptoms of substance abuse and seek professional help for early intervention. In this subchapter, we will explore the importance of seeking professional assistance and how it can positively impact our child's future.

Recognizing the early signs of addiction is the first step towards seeking help. Changes in behavior, sudden mood swings, declining academic performance, withdrawal from family and friends, and unusual secrecy are just a few red flags that could indicate a problem. Rather than ignoring or denying these signs, it is crucial that we take action and reach out to professionals who specialize in addiction prevention and treatment.

By seeking professional help, we can gain a better understanding of our child's situation and the underlying causes of their addiction. Addiction is a complex issue, often influenced by genetic, environmental, and psychological factors. Professionals can conduct thorough assessments and develop personalized treatment plans tailored to our child's unique needs. They can also guide us in creating a supportive and nurturing environment at home, which is essential for the recovery process.

Furthermore, professional intervention can equip us with the knowledge and tools necessary to effectively communicate with our child about addiction. Open and honest conversations are vital in building trust and fostering a healthy relationship. Professionals can guide us in finding the right words, setting boundaries, and offering support without enabling destructive behavior.

Early intervention not only addresses the immediate challenges but also plays a significant role in protecting our child's future. By seeking help early on, we increase the chances of successful recovery and reduce the risk of long-term consequences. Addiction can have devastating effects on various aspects of our child's life, including their physical and mental health, education, relationships, and overall well-being. Seeking professional help empowers us to prevent these consequences from taking hold and allows our child to reclaim their life.

In conclusion, seeking professional help for early intervention is crucial when dealing with addiction in our children. By recognizing the signs, understanding the causes, and obtaining the necessary support, we can play an active role in guiding our child towards recovery and protecting their future. Remember, you are not alone in this journey, and professionals are here to help you navigate the challenges of addiction prevention and treatment. Together, we can make a difference in our children's lives and create a brighter future for them.

Chapter 3: Parenting a Teen with Substance Abuse Problems

Identifying Substance Abuse in Teens

As parents, one of our greatest fears is the possibility of our children falling into the trap of substance abuse. It is crucial to be aware of the signs and symptoms of substance abuse in teenagers, as early intervention can make all the difference in preventing long-term addiction and supporting our children's well-being. In this subchapter, we will explore the key indicators that may signal substance abuse in teens and provide guidance on how parents can address these issues.

The first step in identifying substance abuse in teens is to be aware of changes in their behavior and overall well-being. Look out for sudden changes in their mood, frequent irritability, withdrawal from family and friends, and a decline in academic performance. Additionally, be vigilant about any physical changes such as bloodshot eyes, constant tiredness, unexplained weight loss or gain, and a neglect of personal hygiene.

Communication is vital when dealing with teenagers struggling with substance abuse. It is essential to create an open and non-judgmental environment where your child feels comfortable discussing their concerns. Encourage regular conversations about their day, friends, and any challenges they may be facing. Listen attentively, show empathy, and validate their emotions. By fostering trust and open dialogue, you increase the likelihood of them seeking your guidance and support.

In some cases, professional help may be necessary. If you suspect substance abuse, consider reaching out to a healthcare professional, counselor, or addiction specialist who can provide a comprehensive assessment and guidance on the next steps. Remember, you are not alone in this journey, and seeking professional help is a proactive step towards your child's well-being.

Lastly, prevention is key. Educate yourself and your children about the dangers of substance abuse. Teach them about healthy coping mechanisms, stress management techniques, and the importance of making responsible choices. By instilling strong values, setting clear boundaries, and being actively involved in your child's life, you can reduce the risk of substance abuse.

In conclusion, identifying substance abuse in teens requires vigilance, open communication, and a proactive approach. By being aware of the signs, providing a supportive environment, seeking professional help when needed, and focusing on prevention, we can protect our children's future and help them navigate the challenges of adolescence safely. Remember, your role as a parent is crucial in shaping their understanding of addiction and prevention, and your support can make all the difference in their journey towards a healthy and fulfilling life.

Communicating with a Teenager about Addiction

As parents of young kids, it is crucial to equip ourselves with the necessary knowledge and skills to have open and effective conversations about addiction with our teenagers. Adolescence is a time when they may encounter peer pressure, experimentation, and potential exposure to substances. Therefore, being able to communicate about addiction can greatly contribute to their understanding, prevention, and protection.

When broaching the topic of addiction with your teenager, it is essential to approach the conversation with empathy and understanding. Start by creating a safe and non-judgmental environment where they feel comfortable sharing their thoughts and experiences. Remember, addiction does not discriminate, and even kids from well-rounded families can be susceptible to its grasp.

Begin by discussing the potential risks and consequences associated with substance abuse. Educate them on the impact drugs and alcohol can have on their physical and mental health, relationships, academic performance, and future prospects. Emphasize that addiction is a chronic disease and not a personal failing, ensuring they understand they can reach out for help without shame or stigma.

Encourage open dialogue by actively listening to your teenager's concerns, opinions, and questions. Allow them to express their thoughts and feelings without interruption, and validate their emotions. This approach fosters trust and encourages them to confide in you, which is crucial when addressing addiction-related issues.

It is also important to provide accurate information about addiction. Share stories of recovery and the positive impact of seeking help, as well as the potential consequences of not addressing addiction early on. By providing a balanced understanding, you empower your teenager to make informed decisions and avoid potential pitfalls.

Additionally, emphasize the importance of setting boundaries and making healthy choices. Encourage them to surround themselves with positive influences, engage in hobbies and activities they enjoy, and develop a strong support network of friends and family members. Promote resilience and coping strategies to help them navigate challenges they may face during their teenage years.

Lastly, be a role model by demonstrating responsible behavior and healthy coping mechanisms. Your actions speak louder than words, and your teenager will observe and learn from your approach to stress, emotions, and substance use. Practice open communication within your family, and ensure they feel comfortable seeking your guidance and support when needed.

Communicating with teenagers about addiction can be challenging, but it is an essential conversation to have. By fostering open dialogue, providing accurate information, and being a supportive role model, you play a vital role in preventing addiction in your child's life and protecting their future.

Establishing Rules and Consequences

When it comes to addiction prevention in kids, one of the most crucial aspects is establishing clear rules and consequences. As parents of young kids, it is our responsibility to create a safe and nurturing environment that instills healthy habits and choices in our children. By setting up rules and enforcing them consistently, we can help guide our children towards a future free from addiction.

First and foremost, it is important to establish age-appropriate rules. These rules should reflect your family values and expectations, taking into consideration your child's level of understanding. Make sure to communicate these rules clearly and discuss them with your child, allowing them to have a say and understand the reasoning behind each rule.

Alongside rules, consequences play a vital role in teaching children about accountability. Consequences should be fair and proportional to the rule broken while focusing on teaching rather than punishing. For example, if your child breaks curfew, an appropriate consequence might be to restrict their privileges for a few days. This allows them to learn from their mistakes and understand the importance of following rules.

Consistency is key when it comes to enforcing rules and consequences. Children thrive in a structured environment, knowing what is expected of them and what will happen if they don't comply. By consistently implementing and reinforcing rules, you are teaching your child the importance of boundaries and responsibility.

It is also crucial to lead by example. As parents, we need to demonstrate the behavior we want our children to adopt. If we have rules regarding substance use, such as no smoking or drinking in the house, it is essential that we adhere to these rules ourselves.

By modeling healthy habits and choices, we are providing our children with a strong foundation for making positive decisions in the face of peer pressure.

Remember, establishing rules and consequences is not about control or punishment; it is about protecting our children's future. By setting clear expectations, enforcing consequences, and leading by example, we are equipping our children with the tools they need to navigate the challenges of adolescence and make informed choices regarding substance use.

In the next chapter, we will explore strategies for open communication with your child, fostering trust and understanding, which is another crucial aspect of addiction prevention. Together, we can create a safe and supportive environment that promotes a healthy and addiction-free future for our children.

Supporting Your Teen's Recovery Journey

As parents, we are tasked with the responsibility of guiding our children through life's challenges and ensuring their well-being. However, when it comes to addiction, many parents find themselves at a loss for how to support their teen's recovery journey. In this subchapter, we will provide you with valuable insights and practical strategies to help you navigate this difficult terrain.

Parenting a teenager with substance abuse problems can be an overwhelming experience. It is essential to approach this situation with empathy, understanding, and a non-judgmental attitude. Remember, addiction is a complex disease, and your teen needs your unconditional love and support more than ever.

One of the most crucial aspects of supporting your teen's recovery journey is open and honest communication. Create a safe space for them to share their thoughts and feelings without fear of judgment or punishment. Listen actively and validate their experiences. By doing so, you can help foster a sense of trust and encourage them to seek help when needed.

Educating yourself about addiction and recovery is also vital. Understand the signs and symptoms of substance abuse, as well as the various treatment options available. This knowledge will enable you to make informed decisions and provide the best possible support for your teen.

Nurturing a child with a predisposition to addiction requires a proactive approach. Promote healthy coping mechanisms, such as engaging in physical activities, pursuing hobbies, and fostering strong social connections. Encourage them to develop a strong sense of self-worth and self-esteem, as these factors can serve as protective factors against addiction.

Raising awareness about addiction and prevention in children is an essential step in breaking the cycle of addiction. Engage in open discussions about the risks associated with substance abuse, peer pressure, and the importance of making responsible choices. By fostering a culture of prevention and awareness, you can empower your child to make informed decisions and resist the temptation of drugs and alcohol.

Supporting a loved one through addiction recovery can be emotionally challenging. Encourage them to seek professional help and attend support groups. Remember to prioritize self-care as well, as supporting someone through recovery can take a toll on your own mental and emotional well-being.

In conclusion, supporting your teen's recovery journey requires compassion, understanding, and a commitment to their well-being. By fostering open communication, educating yourself, nurturing resilience, raising awareness, and seeking support, you can provide the necessary support for your teen's recovery journey. Remember, you are not alone in this journey, and there is help available for both you and your teen.

Dealing with Relapses and Setbacks

Relapses and setbacks are a common part of the recovery journey for individuals struggling with addiction. As parents, it can be heartbreaking to witness our children experience these challenges. However, it is crucial to remember that setbacks are not indicative of failure but rather an opportunity for growth and learning.

In this subchapter, we will explore effective strategies for parents of young kids to deal with relapses and setbacks in their children's lives. These tips are not only applicable to those currently struggling with addiction but also beneficial for all parents aiming to prevent addiction and promote a healthy lifestyle.

1. Open Communication: Maintaining an open and non-judgmental line of communication with your child is essential. Encourage them to express their feelings and concerns without fear of punishment or criticism. This will help establish trust, making it easier for them to seek support when facing setbacks.

2. Educate Yourself: Learn about addiction, its signs, and the recovery process. By understanding the challenges your child may encounter, you can provide appropriate support and guidance. Stay updated on the latest research and resources available to help both you and your child through this journey.

3. Seek Professional Help: Reach out to addiction specialists, therapists, or support groups tailored to parents of children struggling with addiction. These professionals can provide valuable guidance and help you navigate the complexities of addiction and relapse prevention.

4. Encourage Healthy Coping Mechanisms: Teach your child alternative ways to cope with stress and negative emotions. Encourage activities such as exercise, creative outlets, and engaging hobbies that promote emotional well-being. By providing healthier coping mechanisms, you can help reduce the likelihood of relapse.

5. Foster a Supportive Environment: Surround your child with a supportive network of family, friends, and mentors who understand the challenges of addiction. Encourage positive influences in their lives and discourage interactions with individuals who may trigger relapse or enable their addictive behaviors.

6. Self-Care: As a parent, it is crucial to prioritize your well-being. Take time for self-care, practice stress-management techniques, and seek support for yourself. By maintaining your own emotional and physical health, you can better support your child through their relapses and setbacks.

Remember, setbacks are a natural part of the recovery process. Rather than viewing them as failures, see them as opportunities for growth and learning. With your unwavering support and the right resources, your child can overcome their setbacks and build a healthier, addiction-free future.

By implementing these strategies, you are taking proactive steps to protect your child's future, promoting addiction prevention, and nurturing their overall well-being.

Chapter 4: Supporting a Loved One through Addiction Recovery

Understanding the Recovery Process

The recovery process for addiction can be complex and challenging, but as parents of young kids, it is crucial to have a thorough understanding of it. In this subchapter, we will delve into the various aspects of the recovery process, including how to support a loved one through addiction recovery, nurturing a child with a predisposition to addiction, and raising awareness about addiction and prevention in children.

Parenting a teen with substance abuse problems is a daunting task, and understanding the recovery process is essential to providing the necessary support. It is important to recognize that recovery is not a linear journey but rather a process that involves ups and downs. By understanding this, parents can better prepare themselves for the challenges that may arise and offer unwavering support to their teen.

Supporting a loved one through addiction recovery requires patience, empathy, and education. By learning about the recovery process, parents can better comprehend the stages their loved one may go through, such as detoxification, therapy, and aftercare. This knowledge enables parents to provide the appropriate support, whether it be emotional, financial, or practical, throughout the recovery journey.

Nurturing a child with a predisposition to addiction requires a proactive approach. Understanding the genetic and environmental factors that contribute to addiction can help parents create a safe and healthy environment for their child. By fostering open communication, setting boundaries, and promoting positive coping mechanisms, parents can empower their child to make healthy choices and reduce the risk of addiction.

Raising awareness about addiction and prevention in children is a crucial step in protecting their future. By educating ourselves and others about the signs and risks of addiction, parents can take proactive measures to prevent substance abuse in their children. This can include teaching them about the dangers of drugs and alcohol, fostering self-esteem and resilience, and promoting healthy coping strategies.

In conclusion, understanding the recovery process is vital for parents of young kids in various situations. Whether they are parenting a teen with substance abuse problems, supporting a loved one through addiction recovery, nurturing a child with a predisposition to addiction, or raising awareness about addiction and prevention in children, having a comprehensive understanding of the recovery process empowers parents to provide the necessary support and make informed decisions.

By equipping ourselves with this knowledge, we can protect our children's future and guide them towards a life free from addiction.

Educating Yourself about Addiction Treatment Options

Subchapter: Educating Yourself about Addiction Treatment Options

As parents, one of our greatest responsibilities is to protect our children from harm. Unfortunately, addiction is a harsh reality that many families face, and it can be devastating for both the individual struggling and their loved ones. However, there is hope. By educating ourselves about addiction treatment options, we can better support our children and provide them with the help they need to overcome this challenging journey.

Understanding the available treatment options is crucial for parents of young kids. Whether you are raising an addict, parenting a teen with substance abuse problems, supporting a loved one through addiction recovery, nurturing a child with a predisposition to addiction, or simply raising awareness about addiction and prevention in children, this knowledge is invaluable.

Firstly, it is essential to recognize that addiction is a complex disease that requires professional help. Treatment options often include a combination of therapy, counseling, and medical intervention. Inpatient or residential treatment programs provide a structured and supportive environment where individuals can focus solely on their recovery. Outpatient programs, on the other hand, offer flexibility for those who require treatment while still maintaining their daily responsibilities.

Behavioral therapy, such as cognitive-behavioral therapy (CBT), has proven to be effective in treating addiction. CBT helps individuals identify and change negative patterns of thinking and behavior, equipping them with healthier coping mechanisms. Family therapy is another vital component, as it addresses the impact of addiction on the entire family unit and fosters healing and understanding.

Medication-assisted treatment (MAT) may also be recommended, particularly for opioid or alcohol addiction. Medications such as methadone, buprenorphine, or naltrexone can help reduce withdrawal symptoms and cravings, allowing individuals to focus on their recovery.

Support groups, such as Alcoholics Anonymous (AA) or Narcotics Anonymous (NA), provide a sense of community and understanding for individuals and their families. These groups offer a safe space for sharing experiences, gaining valuable insights, and building a strong support network.

Educating ourselves about addiction treatment options is not only about finding the right resources for our children but also about understanding how we can provide the necessary support. By staying informed, we can encourage open communication, reduce stigma, and promote a healthier and more compassionate approach to addiction and prevention in children.

Remember, you are not alone in this journey. There are countless resources available, including helplines, support groups, and addiction specialists who can guide you through the process. By educating ourselves and seeking professional help, we can protect our children's future and support them on their path to recovery.

Creating a Supportive Environment at Home

As parents, we play a crucial role in shaping our children's lives and protecting them from the dangers of addiction. One of the most effective ways to prevent addiction in kids is by creating a supportive environment at home. By fostering open communication, setting boundaries, and promoting healthy habits, we can help our children develop the resilience and skills they need to navigate the challenges they may face.

First and foremost, open communication is key. Encourage your children to share their thoughts and feelings without fear of judgment or punishment. Create a safe space where they can talk openly about their experiences, concerns, and pressures they may be facing. Listen attentively and validate their emotions, ensuring they feel heard and understood. By promoting open lines of communication, you can build a trusting relationship that will make it easier for your child to seek guidance and support when needed.

Setting clear boundaries is another essential aspect of creating a supportive environment. Establish rules and expectations that align with your family's values and communicate them consistently. Consistency is key to ensure your child understands the consequences of their actions and feels secure within these boundaries. However, it is important to strike a balance between setting boundaries and allowing your child to make their own choices, as this will help them develop autonomy and decision-making skills.

Promoting healthy habits is also crucial in preventing addiction in kids. Encourage physical activity, a well-balanced diet, and sufficient sleep. These habits not only contribute to overall well-being but also help children develop a sense of self-care and self-discipline. Additionally, educate your child about the risks associated with substance abuse and the importance of making healthy choices for their future.

Lastly, create an atmosphere of understanding and compassion. If you suspect your child may have a predisposition to addiction or if you are already parenting a teen with substance abuse problems, it is essential to approach the issue with empathy and seek professional help. Support groups, therapy, and counseling can provide the guidance and resources needed to navigate these challenging situations.

By creating a supportive environment at home, we can play an active role in preventing addiction in our children. Remember, every child is unique, and the approach may vary depending on their individual needs. By fostering open communication, setting boundaries, promoting healthy habits, and seeking professional help when needed, we can protect our children's future and empower them to make informed choices, leading to a healthier and addiction-free life.

Encouraging Healthy Habits and Activities

In today's fast-paced and technology-driven world, it is crucial for parents to prioritize and encourage healthy habits and activities in their young children. By instilling these habits early on, parents can help protect their children from the risks of addiction later in life. This subchapter aims to provide practical tips and guidance for parents to nurture their children's physical and mental well-being, while promoting addiction prevention.

Creating a healthy lifestyle begins with fostering a positive and supportive environment at home. As parents, it is important to lead by example. Engaging in regular physical activities together as a family, such as going for walks, riding bikes, or playing outdoor games, not only promotes physical health but also strengthens the bond between parents and children.

In addition to physical activities, it is crucial to encourage children to explore a variety of hobbies and interests. This helps them develop a sense of purpose and passion, reducing the likelihood of turning to substance abuse as a means of escape or coping mechanism. Support your child's interests, whether it is art, sports, music, or any other activity that brings them joy and fulfillment.

Furthermore, maintaining open lines of communication is essential. Talk to your children about the dangers of substance abuse in an age-appropriate manner. Educate them on the risks and consequences of addiction, while emphasizing the importance of making healthy choices. Encourage them to express their emotions and concerns, and be attentive and empathetic listeners.

Limiting exposure to media that glamorizes drug and alcohol use is another crucial step. Monitor your child's screen time and ensure they have access to age-appropriate and educational content. Engage in discussions about media portrayals and help them understand the difference between reality and fiction.

Finally, it is vital to create a strong support network for both parents and children. Connect with other parents who share similar concerns and experiences, and seek professional guidance if needed. Remember that addiction prevention is a community effort, and by raising awareness and sharing knowledge, we can help protect our children's future.

By encouraging healthy habits and activities, parents can significantly reduce the risk of addiction in their children. Through open communication, a supportive environment, and a focus on physical and mental well-being, parents can empower their children to make informed and healthy choices, paving the way for a bright and addiction-free future.

Managing Stress and Self-Care as a Supportive Parent

Parenting can be a joyous and rewarding experience, but it can also be incredibly stressful. As parents, we often put our children's needs before our own, neglecting our own well-being in the process. However, it is essential to prioritize self-care and manage stress effectively in order to be a supportive parent and prevent addiction in our children. In this subchapter, we will explore various strategies for managing stress and self-care as a supportive parent.

Stress can have a detrimental impact on our physical and mental health, as well as our ability to be present and attentive parents. Therefore, it is crucial to identify healthy coping mechanisms to reduce stress levels. Engaging in regular physical exercise, such as yoga or walking, can help release tension and improve mood. Additionally, finding time for hobbies or activities that bring joy and relaxation can significantly reduce stress.

Whether it's reading a book, gardening, or painting, these activities can serve as a healthy outlet for stress.

Furthermore, reaching out for support is essential. As parents, we often feel the need to handle everything on our own, but this can lead to burnout and increased stress levels. Building a network of supportive friends and family members who can offer guidance and lend a helping hand can alleviate some of the stress associated with parenting. Additionally, seeking professional help, such as therapy or counseling, can provide valuable tools for managing stress and navigating challenging parenting situations.

Self-care is not selfish; it is a necessary component of being a supportive parent. Taking time for oneself is crucial for recharging and maintaining emotional well-being. Prioritizing self-care can involve simple activities such as taking a bath, practicing mindfulness or meditation, or engaging in activities that bring relaxation and rejuvenation. Remember, by taking care of yourself, you are better equipped to care for your children.

In conclusion, managing stress and practicing self-care are essential aspects of being a supportive parent and preventing addiction in our children. By prioritizing our own well-being, we can model healthy behaviors and create a nurturing environment for our children. Remember that seeking support, engaging in stress-reducing activities, and practicing self-care are not only beneficial for us but also for the overall well-being of our families. Let us prioritize our own mental and emotional health, so we can raise resilient and healthy children.

Chapter 5: Nurturing a Child with Predisposition to Addiction

Genetic Factors and Addiction

Understanding the role of genetic factors in addiction is crucial for parents who are concerned about their children's vulnerability to substance abuse. While it is true that genetics alone does not determine whether someone will become addicted to drugs or alcohol, it does play a significant role in predisposing individuals to addiction. In this subchapter, we will explore how genetic factors can influence addiction and what parents can do to support and protect their children.

Research has shown that there is a genetic component to addiction, with certain individuals having a higher risk due to their family history. If addiction runs in your family, it is important to recognize that your child may have a higher predisposition to developing an addiction. However, it is essential to remember that genetics does not guarantee addiction, and environmental factors also play a significant role.

As a parent, you can play a crucial role in nurturing a child with a predisposition to addiction. Education and open communication are key. By keeping the lines of communication open, you can help your child understand the potential risks they may face and develop healthy coping mechanisms. Encouraging them to express their feelings and emotions in a safe and supportive environment can also be beneficial.

Additionally, raising awareness about addiction and prevention in children is essential. Educate yourself and your child about the dangers of substance abuse, the signs of addiction, and the available resources for help. By being proactive and knowledgeable, you can help your child make informed decisions and support them in making healthier choices.

It is also important to remember that addiction is a disease, and supporting a loved one through addiction recovery can be challenging but necessary. By seeking professional help and joining support groups, you can equip yourself with the tools to better understand addiction and provide the necessary support to your child during their recovery journey.

In conclusion, while genetic factors can contribute to the risk of addiction, they do not determine its outcome. As parents, we have the power to influence and guide our children towards making healthy choices. By raising awareness about addiction, nurturing our children's emotional well-being, and providing support during recovery, we can protect our children's future and prevent addiction in their lives.

Early Intervention Strategies

In this subchapter, we will explore early intervention strategies that can help parents protect their young kids from addiction. As parents, it is crucial to be proactive and vigilant in creating a safe and nurturing environment for our children. By understanding the risk factors and implementing preventive measures early on, we can significantly reduce the likelihood of our children developing addiction problems in the future.

One of the key strategies for early intervention is open communication. Establishing a foundation of trust and creating a safe space for dialogue with our children is essential. Encourage your child to express their thoughts, feelings, and concerns without judgment. By fostering open communication, we can better understand their emotions and address any underlying issues that may contribute to substance abuse later in life.

Another important strategy is education. Educate yourself and your child about the risks and consequences of addiction. Knowledge is power, and by equipping ourselves with information about addiction, we can better recognize warning signs and intervene early. Teach your child about the dangers of substance abuse, the impact it can have on their mental and physical health, as well as the potential legal consequences.

Recognizing the importance of mental health is also crucial in early intervention. Many individuals turn to substances as a means of self-medication for underlying mental health issues. By focusing on nurturing your child's emotional well-being, you can help them develop healthy coping mechanisms and reduce the likelihood of seeking solace in drugs or alcohol. Encourage activities that promote mental health, such as exercise, creative outlets, and spending quality time with loved ones.

Additionally, it is vital to be proactive in identifying and addressing any signs of risk or vulnerability in your child. Certain factors, such as a family history of addiction, can increase the likelihood of substance abuse. By acknowledging these predispositions, you can take appropriate measures to minimize the risks. Seek professional help if necessary, as therapists and counselors can provide valuable guidance and support.

By employing these early intervention strategies, parents can play a pivotal role in protecting their children from addiction. Remember, prevention is always better than cure. By being proactive, educating ourselves and our children, fostering open communication, and addressing any underlying issues, we can create a strong foundation for a healthy and addiction-free future for our kids.

Building Resilience and Protective Factors

In the journey of parenting, one of the most important roles we play is that of protecting our children and preparing them for the challenges they may face in life. As parents of young kids, it is essential for us to understand the significance of building resilience and protective factors in order to prevent addiction in our children. This subchapter will delve into the strategies and approaches that can help nurture a strong foundation of resilience in our kids, equipping them to navigate life's obstacles and make healthy choices.

Resilience acts as a protective shield against the risks and temptations that can lead to addiction. By fostering resilience in our children, we can help them develop the necessary skills and mindset to cope with stress, peer pressure, and adversity. Building resilience starts with creating a nurturing and supportive environment at home. Encouraging open communication, active listening, and providing emotional support will enable our kids to share their feelings and concerns without fear of judgment or punishment.

Another crucial aspect of building resilience is teaching our children healthy coping mechanisms and problem-solving skills. By guiding them in managing their emotions, stress, and conflicts in constructive ways, we empower them to make better choices and develop a sense of self-control. Engaging in activities that promote self-esteem, such as sports, arts, or hobbies, can also contribute to building resilience by instilling a sense of accomplishment and personal growth.

Recognizing the importance of building protective factors is equally essential. Protective factors act as buffers against the risks of addiction. These factors can include strong family bonds, positive peer relationships, meaningful connections with caring adults, and a sense of belonging and purpose. As parents, we can foster these protective factors by fostering healthy relationships within our family, encouraging positive friendships, and involving our children in community activities that promote social connections.

Furthermore, it is crucial to be proactive in educating ourselves and our children about addiction and prevention. By raising awareness about the risks and consequences of substance abuse, we empower our kids to make informed decisions and resist peer pressure. Teaching them about the harmful effects of drugs and alcohol at an early age can help lay the foundation for a healthy, drug-free lifestyle.

In conclusion, building resilience and protective factors in our children is a fundamental aspect of addiction prevention. By creating a nurturing and supportive environment, teaching healthy coping skills, fostering positive relationships, and raising awareness about addiction, we can equip our kids with the tools they need to make healthy choices and navigate life's challenges.

As parents, our role in protecting their future is invaluable, and by focusing on building resilience, we can help them thrive and lead fulfilling, addiction-free lives.

Promoting Healthy Coping Mechanisms

In today's society, where substance abuse and addiction have become prevalent issues, it is crucial for parents to equip their children with healthy coping mechanisms. By doing so, parents can empower their children to navigate life's challenges without resorting to harmful substances. In this subchapter, we will explore various strategies and tools to promote healthy coping mechanisms in children and teenagers.

1. Open and honest communication: Begin by fostering a safe and non-judgmental environment at home. Encourage your children to express their emotions and concerns without fear of punishment or criticism. By openly discussing their feelings, you can guide them towards healthier coping strategies.

2. Teaching emotional intelligence: Help your children identify and understand their emotions. Teach them that it is natural to experience a range of emotions and that each emotion holds valuable information. By recognizing and accepting their feelings, they can learn to cope with them in healthier ways.

3. Encouraging self-care: Teach your children the importance of self-care and self-love. Encourage them to engage in activities that bring them joy and help them relax, such as hobbies, sports, or creative

outlets. By prioritizing self-care, they will learn to manage stress and negative emotions effectively.

4. Building resilience: Life is full of challenges, and resilience is a crucial skill for navigating them. Encourage your children to view setbacks as opportunities for growth and learning. Help them develop problem-solving skills, adaptability, and perseverance, which will enable them to cope with difficult situations without turning to substances.

5. Seeking professional help: If you suspect your child may be struggling with substance abuse or addiction, seek professional help. Addiction is a complex issue that often requires specialized support. Reach out to therapists, counselors, or addiction specialists who can provide guidance and treatment options tailored to your child's needs.

Remember, prevention is always better than cure. By promoting healthy coping mechanisms early on, you can significantly reduce the risk of addiction in your children. Furthermore, educating yourself and others about addiction prevention is vital in raising awareness in your community. Together, we can create a future where children are equipped with the tools they need to thrive, free from the grips of addiction.

Protecting Their Future: A Parent's Guide to Addiction Prevention in Kids is a comprehensive resource that addresses the challenges parents face in raising children amidst the dangers of substance abuse. This book provides practical advice, research-backed strategies, and real-life stories to empower parents in their journey of protecting their children from addiction. Whether you are parenting a young child, a teenager with substance abuse problems, or supporting a loved one through addiction recovery, this guide will offer valuable insights and tools to help you navigate the complex world of addiction prevention.

Seeking Professional Guidance for Parenting Challenges

Parenting is a journey filled with joy, love, and countless challenges. As parents of young kids, we want nothing more than to protect and guide our children towards a bright and successful future. However, when faced with the daunting task of raising a child who may be at risk for addiction or is already struggling with substance abuse, we may feel overwhelmed and unsure of how to best support them.

In times like these, seeking professional guidance is crucial. It is important to remember that you are not alone in this journey. There are experts and professionals who specialize in addiction prevention, substance abuse treatment, and parenting techniques that can help you navigate through these challenges.

When it comes to raising a child with a predisposition to addiction, seeking professional guidance can provide you with the tools and knowledge necessary to create a safe and supportive environment. Professionals can assist you in understanding the warning signs, developing prevention strategies, and implementing effective communication techniques to foster a healthy relationship with your child.

For parents who are dealing with a teen struggling with substance abuse problems, professional guidance can be a lifeline. Addiction is a complex issue, and it requires specialized treatment and support. Professionals can help you find appropriate treatment programs, provide counseling for both the teen and the family, and offer guidance on how to navigate the recovery process.

Supporting a loved one through addiction recovery can be emotionally challenging and exhausting. Seeking professional guidance can provide you with the necessary tools to cope with your own emotions, set healthy boundaries, and offer the support your loved one needs to maintain their recovery.

Additionally, raising awareness about addiction and prevention in children is vital. Professionals can guide you on how to educate your child about the dangers of substance abuse, equip them with refusal skills, and foster a resilient mindset to navigate peer pressure.

Remember, seeking professional guidance does not mean you are failing as a parent. It shows that you are proactive, committed, and willing to do whatever it takes to protect your child's future. There are resources available that can provide you with the support and knowledge you need to navigate these challenges successfully.

In conclusion, seeking professional guidance for parenting challenges related to addiction prevention, substance abuse, and recovery is essential. Professionals can offer valuable insights, effective strategies, and emotional support that can help you navigate through these complex issues. By seeking their expertise, you are taking a proactive step towards protecting your child's future and ensuring their well-being. Remember, you don't have to face these challenges alone. Help is available, and together we can create a safe and nurturing environment for our children.

Chapter 6: Raising Awareness about

Addiction and Prevention in Children

Educating Yourself and Others about Addiction

As parents, it is crucial for us to be well-informed about addiction and its potential impact on our children. By educating ourselves and others about addiction, we can take proactive measures to protect our kids from falling into its grasp. In this subchapter, we will delve into the importance of understanding addiction, how to educate ourselves and our children about it, and ways to raise awareness in our communities.

To effectively prevent addiction, we must first understand its root causes and risk factors. By familiarizing ourselves with the science behind addiction, we can better comprehend the complexities of this disease. The more we know about the genetic, environmental, and psychological factors that contribute to addiction, the better equipped we are to identify potential warning signs in our children.

Once we have educated ourselves about addiction, it becomes our responsibility to pass on this knowledge to our children. Open and honest conversations about drugs, alcohol, and their potential consequences should start at an early age. By fostering a safe environment for discussion, we can help our kids make informed decisions and resist peer pressure.

Supporting a loved one through addiction recovery can be an immensely challenging journey. This subchapter will provide guidance on how to navigate this process, offering tips on effective communication, setting boundaries, and accessing professional help. By equipping ourselves with the necessary tools, we can become a pillar of strength for our loved ones as they strive towards recovery.

Some children may have a predisposition to addiction due to genetic factors or family history. For these kids, it is essential to provide extra support and nurture their emotional well-being. This subchapter will explore ways to create a nurturing environment, including fostering strong relationships, promoting healthy coping mechanisms, and encouraging self-esteem and resilience.

Lastly, raising awareness about addiction and prevention in children is vital in our communities. By actively participating in local initiatives, events, and workshops, we can help break the stigma surrounding addiction and educate others about its dangers. This subchapter will provide resources and ideas for organizing awareness campaigns, engaging with schools and community organizations, and advocating for addiction prevention programs.

In conclusion, educating ourselves and others about addiction is crucial in protecting our children's future. By understanding addiction, having open conversations with our kids, supporting loved ones through recovery, nurturing those with a predisposition, and raising awareness in our communities, we can create a safe and informed environment that reduces the risk of addiction in our kids. Together, we can make a difference and ensure a brighter future for our children.

Talking to Other Parents and Community Members

As parents, we often find ourselves navigating the challenging terrain of raising our children in a world filled with potential pitfalls and dangers. When it comes to addiction prevention in kids, it is essential to remember that we are not alone in this journey. By reaching out to other parents and community members, we can create a network of support that will not only benefit our own children but also contribute to raising awareness about addiction prevention.

One of the most effective ways to tackle addiction prevention is by engaging in open and honest conversations with other parents. By sharing our concerns, experiences, and strategies, we can learn from one another and gain valuable insights into effective prevention techniques. Whether it's discussing how to talk to our children about the dangers of substance abuse or sharing resources and information, these conversations can be instrumental in creating a united front against addiction.

Community involvement is another crucial aspect of addiction prevention. By actively participating in community events and initiatives, we can raise awareness about addiction and prevention in children. Collaborating with local schools, organizations, and healthcare professionals can help us organize workshops, seminars, and awareness campaigns to educate parents and community members about the risks and warning signs of addiction. Together, we can create a supportive environment that fosters healthy habits and discourages substance abuse.

In addition to supporting our own children, it is important to extend our compassion and understanding to parents who are facing the challenges of parenting a teen with substance abuse problems. By listening without judgment and offering support, we can help these parents navigate the difficult journey of recovery. Sharing our own experiences and resources can provide them with the tools they need to support their loved ones through addiction recovery.

Furthermore, nurturing a child with a predisposition to addiction requires a unique approach. Connecting with other parents who have similar experiences can provide a sense of community and understanding. By learning about therapeutic techniques, counseling options, and creating a safe and supportive environment, we can help our children thrive despite their predisposition.

It is crucial to recognize that addiction prevention is not the sole responsibility of parents. By actively engaging with other parents and community members, we can create a powerful force that advocates for addiction prevention in children. By sharing information, supporting one another, and raising awareness, we can protect our children's future and create a community that prioritizes their well-being. Together, we can make a difference in the lives of our children and future generations.

Advocating for Addiction Prevention Programs in Schools

When it comes to protecting our children from the dangers of addiction, parents play a crucial role. While much of the responsibility lies within the confines of our own homes, there is also a need to advocate for addiction prevention programs in schools. By advocating for these programs, we can ensure that our children receive the education and support they need to make informed decisions about substance abuse.

One of the key reasons to advocate for addiction prevention programs in schools is the fact that prevention is always better than cure. By providing children with the necessary tools and knowledge about the risks associated with substance abuse, we can empower them to make healthier choices. These programs can teach them about the dangers of drugs and alcohol, as well as offer strategies for resisting peer pressure and building resilience.

Moreover, addiction prevention programs in schools can help parents identify warning signs of substance abuse. By learning about the signs and symptoms of addiction, parents can intervene early and seek appropriate help for their children. These programs can also provide resources and referral information for parents who may be struggling to navigate the challenges of parenting a teen with substance abuse problems.

Advocating for addiction prevention programs in schools is also crucial for fostering a supportive community. By raising awareness about addiction and prevention in children, we can reduce the stigma associated with substance abuse. This can create an environment where parents feel comfortable seeking help for their children, and where children feel supported in their journey towards recovery.

Furthermore, advocating for addiction prevention programs in schools is especially important for parents who are raising a child with a predisposition to addiction. These programs can offer specialized support and guidance to help parents navigate the unique challenges they may face. By equipping parents with the knowledge and resources they need, we can increase the chances of preventing addiction and promoting healthy behaviors in these children.

In conclusion, advocating for addiction prevention programs in schools is an essential step in protecting our children's future. By providing them with the necessary education, support, and resources, we can empower them to make informed decisions and resist the temptations of substance abuse. As parents, it is our responsibility to raise awareness, advocate for these programs, and ensure the well-being of our children. Together, we can create a safer and healthier environment for our kids.

Organizing Awareness Events and Workshops

As parents, we play a vital role in equipping our children with the knowledge and skills they need to make healthy choices, especially when it comes to addiction prevention. One powerful way to do this is by organizing awareness events and workshops within our community. These events have the potential to make a significant impact not only on our own children but also on other families facing similar challenges. In this subchapter, we will explore the importance of organizing such events and provide practical tips on how to make them successful.

Awareness events and workshops serve as a platform to educate parents, caregivers, and community members about the risks and consequences of addiction in children. By raising awareness, we can empower parents with the necessary tools to recognize the signs of substance abuse and intervene early on. It also offers an opportunity for parents to share their experiences, offer support, and learn from one another.

To organize a successful awareness event or workshop, start by identifying the specific topics and themes that are most relevant to your audience. Consider inviting experts in the field of addiction prevention, such as counselors, psychologists, or recovering addicts, to share their insights and provide valuable guidance. Additionally, reach out to local organizations that focus on addiction prevention or recovery to collaborate and share resources.

Promoting the event is crucial to ensure a good turnout. Utilize various communication channels, such as social media, local newspapers, and community bulletin boards, to spread the word. Creating visually appealing flyers or posters can also help grab people's attention and generate interest.

During the event, engage participants through interactive activities and discussions. Provide practical strategies and tools that parents can implement at home to prevent addiction in their children. Encourage open dialogue and create a safe space for parents to ask questions and seek advice.

Remember that organizing a single event may not be enough. Consider establishing an ongoing support group or workshop series to continue the conversation and provide ongoing support to parents and families dealing with addiction-related issues.

By organizing awareness events and workshops, we can come together as a community to protect our children's future. Together, we can raise awareness about addiction prevention in children, offer support to those in need, and ultimately create a safer and healthier environment for our families.

Supporting Local Addiction and Recovery Organizations

One of the most effective ways for parents to actively participate in addiction prevention and recovery is by supporting local addiction and recovery organizations. These organizations play a crucial role in creating awareness, providing resources, and offering support to individuals and families dealing with addiction. By getting involved, parents can not only help their own children but also contribute to the well-being of the entire community.

Local addiction and recovery organizations offer a range of services that can be beneficial for parents of young kids. They often organize educational programs and workshops that provide valuable information about addiction prevention, signs of substance abuse, and effective communication techniques. Attending these events can equip parents with the necessary knowledge and tools to identify and address potential addiction issues in their children.

Additionally, these organizations can connect parents with support groups where they can interact with other parents facing similar challenges. Sharing experiences, struggles, and strategies can provide a sense of solidarity and comfort, alleviating the feelings of isolation that often accompany parenting a child with addiction or substance abuse problems.

Supporting local addiction and recovery organizations not only helps parents personally but also contributes to the broader goal of raising awareness about addiction and prevention in children. By actively participating in fundraisers, volunteering, or donating to these organizations, parents can help them continue their important work in the community. This support enables organizations to reach more families, provide counseling services, and develop prevention programs tailored to the needs of children and teens.

Furthermore, parents can play an active role in nurturing a child with a predisposition to addiction by seeking guidance and advice from these organizations. They often have professional staff members who can provide insights and strategies for creating a supportive and healthy environment for children at risk.

In conclusion, supporting local addiction and recovery organizations is a vital step in addiction prevention and recovery for parents of young kids. By engaging with these organizations, parents can access valuable resources, gain knowledge, find support, and contribute to raising awareness about addiction in children. Together, we can create a safer and healthier future for our children and communities.

Conclusion: Empowering Parents to Protect Their Children's Future

In today's fast-paced and complicated world, parents face numerous challenges when it comes to raising their children. As parents of young kids, it is crucial that we equip ourselves with the necessary knowledge and tools to protect our children from the dangers of addiction. Throughout this book, we have explored the various aspects of addiction prevention in kids and how we can actively play a role in safeguarding their future.

Raising an addict is an unimaginable nightmare for any parent. However, by being proactive and attentive, we can create a nurturing environment that reduces the risk of our children falling into the trap of addiction. By setting clear boundaries, establishing open lines of communication, and providing a supportive and loving home, we lay the foundation for a healthy and addiction-free future for our children.

Parenting a teen with substance abuse problems can be an incredibly challenging experience. It is essential to approach this situation with empathy, understanding, and a commitment to seeking professional help. By educating ourselves about addiction, attending support groups, and accessing the right resources, we can navigate this difficult journey together with our child, helping them find the path to recovery and healing.

Supporting a loved one through addiction recovery requires patience, compassion, and unwavering support. As parents, we have a unique position to provide the love and encouragement needed during this challenging time. By educating ourselves about addiction, attending family therapy sessions, and seeking guidance from addiction specialists, we can play a crucial role in our loved one's recovery journey.

Nurturing a child with a predisposition to addiction requires a proactive and preventative approach. By implementing healthy coping mechanisms, promoting emotional intelligence, and fostering a sense of belonging and self-worth, we empower our children to make informed and responsible choices. Early intervention and open conversations about the risks and consequences of addiction can significantly reduce their vulnerability.

Raising awareness about addiction and prevention in children is a responsibility that falls on all parents. By engaging in community initiatives, supporting addiction education programs, and speaking openly about the topic, we can break the stigma surrounding addiction and create a supportive environment for those affected. By sharing our knowledge and experiences, we can empower other parents to take proactive steps in protecting their children's future.

In conclusion, as parents, we have a unique opportunity and responsibility to protect our children from the devastating effects of addiction. By educating ourselves, seeking support, and fostering a nurturing and communicative environment, we can empower our children to make healthy choices and lead fulfilling lives free from the grip of addiction. Let us take the necessary steps today to safeguard our children's future and create a society that prioritizes addiction prevention in kids.